D0987643

A Woman's Guide to De-Stress for Success:

10 Essential Tips to Conquer Stress & Live at Your Best

By

Dr. Tiffany Lowe-Payne

A Woman's Guide to De-Stress for Success:
10 Essential Tips to Conquer Stress & Live at Your Best

Dr. Tiffany Lowe-Payne

ISBN: 0997358017
ISBN-13: 978-0997358018

Dr. Tiffany Lowe-Payne

Bringing Out Your Best: Mind, Body & Spirit!

Beloved, I wish above all things that thou mayest prosper and be in health, even as thy soul prospereth.

3 John 1:2, KJV

To my mother, who made so many sacrifices as she showed her children unconditional love; and who instilled in me the belief that my life would be used for a cause greater than myself, I dedicate this book to you.

Testimonials

"Dr. Tiffany Lowe-Payne's book is amazing! It's a needed reminder of how chronic stress can affect our health if we're not careful. She offers practical tools to make it better. This book is an essential tool for every Type A workaholic, including myself, to get their stress under control before it's too late!"
- Myla Bennett, MD, plastic surgeon & beauty preservation strategist™
Founder and CEO, Ederra Bella Plastic Surgery & Med Spa, Inc.

"A Woman's Guide to De-Stress for Success" provides an inspirational game plan for stress management. Dr. Lowe-Payne's use of her medical expertise in combination with her beautiful spirit and obvious passion for helping others makes this book a must-read for every woman coping with the demands of everyday life!"
- Carol Gibbs, MD, psychiatrist
Owner and CEO, Senior Health and Education Partners, PLLC

"I am excited to see Dr. Tiffany's first book get into the hands of women who are ready to 'de-stress' and begin to live their lives as we are meant to live – victoriously! Every woman carries the key to success within. Dr. Tiffany helps you to find and use that key to your advantage to obtain optimal health. Be prepared to get healthy from the inside out!"
- Charlotte Paolini, DO, family practice
Chair, Department of Family Medicine Campbell University, School of Osteopathic Medicine

"A Woman's Guide to De-Stress for Success" is an amazing tool for women who lead busy lives, to learn practical tips to 'de-stress' and live at their best! If you're looking for a guide that will not only be inspiring but will help to transform your life for the better, then this book is just for you!"
- Dineen Merriweather, marketing director and event specialist, Radio One, Inc.

"This is a must-read for every woman, especially working moms. Being a wife and mom of two with a full-time job and a rising business, "A Woman's Guide to De-Stress for Success" was exactly what the doctor ordered. A great guide to finding that inner peace, both physically and spiritually, to keep us moving toward our victory in life. In short… this is exactly what I needed right now!"
- Melissa Wade-Cutler, Wade In The Water, LLC radio personality, The Light 103.9 FM

"Finally, a book has been written to help women de-stress while moving toward wholeness! Dr. Tiffany has successfully combined medical science with key daily activities to help any woman deal with stress. "A Woman's Guide to De-Stress for Success" is transparent and practical, and will give you what you need to move forward physically and emotionally. All women should read this book and adhere to its recommendations. You will indeed be de-stressed!"
- Dr. Saundra Wall-Williams, Ph.D., founder, Vision Building Institute for Women

Important Note to Readers

The information contained in this book is for informational and educational purposes only. It is not intended to give personalized diagnosis, treatment or cure for any medical conditions that you may have, nor is it meant to be a substitute for personal medical advice, diagnosis or treatment that you have received from your doctor, therapist or other healthcare provider. Please do not disregard the medical advice, or delay seeking treatment from your healthcare provider based on any information that you have obtained in this book.

It is also important to obtain proper medical advice by seeking the counsel of your personal physician or other licensed healthcare professional prior to making any changes to your lifestyle or healthcare plan based on the information that you've received in this book.

Special Thanks

Contributor:
Natasha T. Brown

Editor:
Mira Lowe

Cover Photographer:
Douglas Everett Payne

Cover Design & Layout:
Brown & Duncan Brand, LLC.

Publishing & Research:
The Institute of Transformational
Health & Wellness Inc.

Dr. Tiffany Lowe-Payne

CONTENTS

Share your thoughts with Dr. Tiffany Lowe-Payne about "A Woman's Guide to De-Stress for Success." Send a tweet to @DrLowePayne with the hashtag #DeStressForSuccess. You may also "Ask Dr. Tiffany" medical-related questions and learn more about The Institute of Transformational Health & Wellness at DrTiffanyLowePayne.com

ACKNOWLEDGMENTS

When striving to achieve your dreams, there are those who believe in your vision as much as you do, and those who stand in the gap to lend a helping hand so that you can succeed. To all of you who believed in me and this project, and who never let me fall, I want to sincerely thank you.

I would like to give special acknowledgements to my coach, Dr. Saundra Wall-Williams, who helped me to understand the vision that God gave me to share with the world. I also want to thank Natasha Brown and Melisa Duncan of Brown & Duncan Brand, LLC, for bringing my vision to life. You saw the dream in my heart and helped me to portray it in such an eloquent way that I pray will be a blessing to all who read this work.

To my family, biological and spiritual, who have always believed in me and continually encouraged me to reach for the stars as you've offered valuable advice, wisdom and unwavering support, thank you so much for your love. I am truly grateful for each of you and I know that I would not have achieved all that I've accomplished in life without you as the wind beneath my wings. I want to give special thanks to my five brothers — Herbert Lowe, Jr., Curtis Lowe, Nolan Lowe, Lamonte Lowe and Brent Lowe — who along with our mother have always been my biggest sources of strength and guidance. As the youngest of the bunch, I have looked to you as role models and am extremely grateful for the love and counsel that you have given me. To the sisters that God has allowed me to have through marriage, Mira, Arlene and Renarda, thank you for being strong virtuous women of purpose, who are not only full of wisdom and grace but who I can always count on for laughter, encouragement, advice and genuine love. Mira, I am so grateful for your selfless heart as you gave of your time and expertise to help me with this book. You saw the passion in my heart and committed yourself to helping me make this a success. Thank you!

To my circle of trust — the girlfriends that I've been blessed to have over the years who have stood by me along the way and support me in this season as I strive to inspire other women to live at their best — I love and appreciate you. Special thanks to my dearest friends Tamara Turman and Francoise Desir, who have believed in me and my vision from the very beginning and kept me accountable to my mission and purpose. Also, thank you to my friend and attorney, Geneva Yourse, who has not only been a great source of support, but who uses her wisdom and expertise to ensure that my dreams are protected.

I also want to acknowledge my husband, Douglas, who is not only the love of my life but my best friend. You have supported me wholeheartedly along this journey and I am so grateful that God placed us together as partners for life. For your dedication and love, I want to say thank you. And to my two boys, Andre' and Jordan, I love you with all of my heart. God truly blessed us when He gave us each of you. I look forward to seeing the men you will become and I am grateful for the success that I know you are predestined for.

To all of the women whom I have treated over the years, especially the ones who came to me in a state of brokenness and allowed me to help them become whole, I want to give you a special thanks. You are truly the inspiration for this book and have helped me to realize the gift that God has given me to inspire women to live at their best. I am truly humbled that you have trusted me with your health and welfare. I am committed to continuing to use this platform to encourage and inspire the lives of countless others.

To God — the first love of my life; the one who protects me and who has showered me with an abundance of blessings — I give you all the glory. Thank you for placing this vision inside of me and for using me as a vessel to spread your joy. I pray you will sanction this work and that all who read it will be blessed as they sense your love and your presence. Transform their lives for the better, in a way unlike ever before –Amen.

Introduction

Welcome to the *best* days of the rest of your life! By deciding to read this book, you have made an awesome choice to take control of your health and begin to reclaim the whole you. I am confident that if you read this entire book and apply the lessons presented, you will be on your way to living happier and healthier as you travel on the road to your destiny. For that, I congratulate you! Now, let's start your journey to total transformation!

Have you ever uttered the words, *"I've been under a lot of stress lately?"* If you are like most people, no doubt that you have. In today's world full of daily tasks, deadlines and demands, feeling stressed is so common that it has become a part of our definition of normal. If you've ever felt over-whelmed, unsettled, under pressure, tense or anxious when faced with a challenge or new endeavor, then you have experienced stress. But, before we jump into my *10 Tips to De-Stress for Success,* I want to dispel a myth that you have probably been led to believe — that all stress is bad. Not true! According to Hans Selye, MD (an endocrinologist who coined the term "stress" and was the first to identify how it affects the body in 1932), stressors actually come from good (*Eustress*) or bad (*Distress*) circumstances, thus producing positive or negative results. When it comes to your health, your body cannot distinguish a good stressor from a bad one. All it knows is that it is being taken out of its norm and considers any stressor to be a potential threat. Therefore, it reacts by releasing the same cascade of hormones no matter what. These hormones include **norepinephrine, adrenaline** and **cortisol** — the primary stress hormones — which can affect your body in many ways. In the short term, stress hormones can be quite beneficial as they help you to stay more alert, focused and ready to tackle problems head on. However, if you stay in crisis mode for too long, those same hormones can become detrimental and cause you to have significant health issues as chronic stress can impact almost every organ system within our bodies.

Take a look at the following list of symptoms and diseases associated with chronic stress. Are you experiencing any of these?

(See Table 1: Manifestations of Chronic Stress. Copyright 2016 The Institute of Transformational Health and Wellness, Inc. All Rights Reserved.)

Manifestations of Chronic Stress

<u>Cognitive Symptoms:</u>	<u>Emotional Symptoms:</u>
• Memory impairment or loss • Inability to focus or concentrate • Racing thought processes • Irrational thoughts or paranoia • Cynical or negative thoughts	• Anxiety/panic attacks • Excessive worry • Short-tempered • Feeling overwhelmed • Depression/loss of interest • Increased irritability or agitation
<u>Physical Symptom/Diagnoses:</u>	<u>Behavioral Symptoms:</u>
• Aches and pains (i.e. chest, headache, fibromyalgia) • Abdominal symptoms (i.e. irritable bowel, reflux, ulcers) • Insomnia • Decreased libido • Excessive fatigue • Decreased immune system (frequent colds) • Weight gain or loss • High blood pressure • Diabetes • Increased asthma attacks • Heart palpitations or disease • Stroke	• Change in eating habits (too much or too little, emotional eating) • Sleeping disturbance • Emotional lability (mood swings) • Procrastination or neglect • Frequent complaining • Nervous habits (i.e. biting nails, twitching, restless legs) • Self-medicating (alcohol, drugs, food, excessive shopping) • "Acting out" or "high-risk" behaviors

It is important to realize that not everyone handles stress in the same manner. Some people can manage it very well and function at high levels during periods of extreme stress, while others cannot. With that being said, no one can stay in "Energizer Bunny" mode or constant flurry forever. If left unchecked, "busyness" can lead to people feeling overwhelmed and they will eventually burn out. That is why it's vital to regularly manage your stress. In this book, I will show you how to apply simple techniques to your daily regimen that will lower your stress level and help you stay on top of your game! You may have heard of some of these tips before, but I would like to take it a step further by explaining the scientific and spiritual principles behind them and show you how mastering these concepts can improve your life. I encourage you to carry this guide in your handbag or briefcase as a reminder of the importance of lowering your stress. Use it throughout the day, as a workbook, to take notes and reflect on ways that you can de-stress so that you can perform at your best!

Now, I am a firm believer that positive thoughts in the morning can set the tone for your entire day. A vital precursor to managing your stress is to command your mornings by establishing a healthy routine. When counseling patients in my office, I can often pinpoint how and where their stress began. So, I will ask you one of the first questions that I ask them: *What are the first things that you see, touch, hear, think or do each morning?* For most people, their cell phone is somewhere in that mix — a habit that many mistakenly think is harmless. If this sounds familiar, consider this — each time when you wake up and the first thing that you lay your eyes on is an alarming text message, email or social media post, how does it make you feel? I am willing to bet that it disturbs your peace and may even have an adverse effect on your whole day!

Break the cycle of anxiety and negativity by starting your day with positive thinking. Command your mornings by not allowing unwanted stress to be the first thing that you experience at the onset of a brand new day. We will talk in more detail about this in Tip 6.

You are almost ready to begin the journey of de-stressing your life.

It is very important to me that I live by example in order to help others do the same. As a result, the advice shared in the following pages are strategies that I have learned to implement in my own life and work. Once I learned the alarming fact, that over 75 percent of Americans report having at least one symptom of stress within the last month and 42 percent say that they have engaged in unhealthy behaviors because of stress, I knew stress management had to be an integral part of my medical practice. My passion is to help women who feel broken become whole. This isn't just limited to my patients but to anyone who feels overwhelmed, overburdened and looking for a better way. I am a doctor with a heart for people and feel called to empower you to become healthier. That starts with helping you remove some of the stress out of your life!

You may ask what makes this book different from any other book about stress? The answer is simple. As a doctor, I want you to understand not only *what* to do but *why*. When people understand why healthcare providers make certain recommendations, they are more motivated to take an active role in the management of their medical problems. This often significantly improves the quality of their health and the success of the treatment plan that their clinician prescribes. In addition, as a woman of great faith, I also believe that it is extremely important for you to understand how exercising your faith when needed has been scientifically proven to lower your stress level and give you a greater sense of well-being. And to help further this point, I use my own life experiences as examples! So, consider this as a partnership between us. I want you to be knowledgeable and feel confident to make healthy decisions to live at your best — mind, body and spirit!

Now are you ready? Let's get started!

TIP 1: IDENTIFY THE PROBLEM: "THE STRESS TEST"

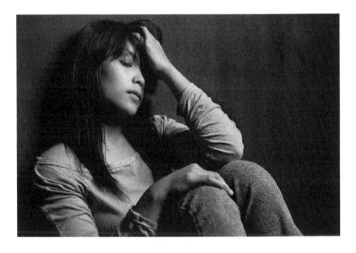

If you want to "de-stress" your life, first recognize that you are indeed stressed.

It sounds like a simple concept, but at times realizing that you are stressed is hard because you can easily get caught up in being "busy." We can also be driven by our human nature to be "fixers." That means when we are presented with a problem or task, we naturally want to help find a solution. This is especially true for women because we are natural multi-taskers and nurturers. However, if you continue to add more to your plate when you are already busy, you will eventually become overwhelmed. It is essential to be in tune with your body so that when you begin to feel pressured, you can take a step back, reprioritize and refocus.

I began to teach on stress management after seeing so many women who appear to have it together on the outside, but who are broken in pieces on the inside. They seem to be doing well in their role(s) as super-moms, faithful friends and loving companions. Some have even reached high levels in their careers as managers, directors and presidents/CEOs of their own companies. In every sense of the word, they are successful. But when they come to see me and talk about the daily issues that they are dealing with, they are actually overburdened and stressed! These women often come in wanting some type of explanation or medication for the symptoms that they are experiencing including migraines, stomach pains, sleepless nights, weight gain, heart palpitations, irritability, anxiety — you name it! (See Table 1.) After I ask them a series of questions to determine the root cause of why they are feeling this way, they often realize with tears in their eyes that they are just stressed out. As pointed out earlier, over 75 percent of Americans say they have recently experienced stress. What is more striking — women actually report having higher stress levels than men. This is especially true for women who are married, those who are parents or millennials (those born between 1980-mid 2000s). All of these groups report higher levels of stress when compared to the rest of Americans surveyed. In addition, studies have shown that although approximately 40 percent of women report that their stress levels have increased over the last year, many also admit that they have not had an open discussion with their healthcare provider about lowering it. The good news is that stress-related disease can be prevented. The first step is to recognize the signs, then you will be able to set a plan in motion to do something about it.

Dr. Tiffany's Pearl of Wisdom:

Don't be too "busy" trying to be the Jack or Jackie of all trades. Become the master of a few! Learn to delegate and set boundaries for the people and roles that you manage.

Before moving on to Tip 2, take a moment to "test" your stress. **Are you experiencing any of the symptoms that we have mentioned so far?** Answer the following questions to assess how you are feeling and if you may be dealing with the effects of chronic stress.

Dr. Tiffany's Stress Level Assessment

Answer all the questions and then add up the points to get your score on how you're managing stress.

1. **Do you have difficulty remembering things, staying focused on tasks or procrastinate often?**
    a) No, I'm always laser focused. (0 points)
    b) Sometimes, but I'm usually able to get things done. (1 point)
    c) Yes, I have issues with one of these and often need reminders to get things done. (2 points)

2. **Do you find that you are easily irritated by people or when things don't go your way?**
    a) No, I am usually even tempered. (0 points)
    b) Sometimes I get irritated, but calm easily. (1 point)
    c) Yes, I must admit that I often get upset, even at little things. (2 points)

3. **Do you feel exhausted by the end of your day?**
    a) No, I usually feel pretty good and have a lot of energy. (0 points)
    b) On occasion, however this is not a regular occurrence. (1 point)
    c) Absolutely! My day is very busy and I am worn out by bedtime. (2 points)

4. Do you get at least 6 hours of quality sleep each night?

    a)   Yes, I sleep very well and wake up feeling refreshed. (0 points)

    b)   Sometimes, although I may have nights where I have difficulty sleeping. (1 point)

    c)   No, I have trouble falling asleep or staying asleep and often lie awake if I do not take something. (2 points)

5. How often do you feel that you are stretched too thin?

    a)   Rarely. (0 points)

    b)   Occasionally, but these are on limited occasions. (1 point)

    c)   I like to make people happy, so I often find that I have a lot on my plate. (2 points)

6. Do you exercise regularly?

    a)   Yes, I exercise at least 3 days a week. (0 points)

    b)   I work out occasionally, but I can't say that I exercise on a regular basis. (1 point)

    c)   I don't have time to exercise. (2 points)

7. Do you have issues with acid reflux, irritable bowel syndrome or stomach ulcers?

    a)   No, I do not have any stomach issues. (0 points)

    b)   I have occasional issues with reflux, but this is not on a regular basis. (1 point)

    c)   Yes, I frequently have stomach problems and have to take meds to help with my symptoms. (2 points)

8. Do you find that you smoke, have a drink, or go shopping to help relieve stress?
   a)   No. (0 points)
   b)   I do at times but not regularly. (1 point)
   c)   Yes, I do one of these things regularly as my vice to relieve stress. (2 points)

9. Do you have issues with feeling depressed, anxious or generally unhappy?
   a)   No. (0 points)
   b)   I feel down or anxious at times, but I am usually okay. (1 point)
   c)   Yes, I must admit that I have been feeling down or anxious and need help. (2 points)

10. How often do you find yourself snacking or eating unhealthy foods when you are not hungry as a response to stress or feeling emotional?
   a)   Rarely, I try to maintain a healthy diet. (0 points)
   b)   I binge occasionally but I don't make a habit of it. (1 point)
   c)   I have to admit that I am an emotional eater and use food to help me feel better. (2 points)

11. How often do you do things to pamper yourself?
   a)   I make a regular habit to take time to rejuvenate myself. (0 points)
   b)   Sometimes, but I could do better. (1 point)
   c)   Rarely, I wish I could but I don't have time. (2 points)

12. How often do you pray or meditate?

   a)   All the time! I make it a regular part of my daily routine. (0 points)

   b)   I do sometimes, but I could do better. (1 point)

   c)   I do not pray or meditate on any regular basis. (2 points)

13. Do you feel cynical about your job?

   a)   No, I love my job! (0 points)

   b)   At times, but I generally do not have a problem with my job. (1 point)

   c)   Yes, I often complain about my job, and would love to change what I do for a living. (2 points)

14. Are you a workaholic?

   a)   No, I work a fixed schedule and have no problem leaving at quitting time. (0 points)

   b)   I stay at work sometimes to catch up on things, but try not to make it a habit. (1 point)

   c)   Yes, I have trouble putting work down and often work extended hours. (2 points)

15. Do you have a good support system of family and friends?

   a)   Yes, I have many people who I can talk to. (0 points)

   b)   I have some friends, but do not always feel comfortable talking to them. (1 point)

   c)   No, I usually handle things on my own. (2 points)

Assessment: Total Possible Points = 30

0-5 points Green Zone: You are doing a wonderful job of controlling your stress. Keep up the great work!

6-15 points Yellow Zone: You are experiencing some of the symptoms that are associated with chronic stress. This can affect your health if you allow your stress level to stay elevated for too long. Keep reading this book and learn practical tips to easily lower your stress level and live a balanced lifestyle.

15 points Red (Danger) Zone: You are at serious risk for major health issues that are secondary to experiencing chronic stress. This book will definitely help you with some important tips, but it is also vital that you seek the advice of a licensed healthcare professional who can help you come up with a personalized plan for better health.

How did you fair?

Are you at risk for developing health issues as a result of your stress level?
As you continue to read this book, I encourage you to take an honest look at your lifestyle and assess where you can make adjustments.
I have included some questions and exercises to help you along the way. I have also included some "Personal Reflections" pages for you to take notes as you reflect on your thoughts and plans.

Use this as a workbook to create a concrete plan and begin to "De-Stress for Success!"

TIP 2: BE STILL

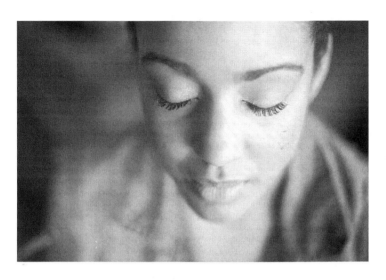

Once you recognize that you're stressed, take a step back, get still and refocus.

"It is in those times when we are still and quiet, that we hear our greatest voice." ~ Dr. Tiffany

Have you ever been so consumed with the daily demands of life that you have felt as though your energy levels were completely depleted? If you have answered yes to this question, take comfort you are not alone. In our modern society where the expectation is to continually strive for success no matter what, you can easily become swamped by all of the things which may cause you to lose focus on what is most important if you are not careful— your well-being. As you are going through your day tackling problems and tasks at record pace, it is critical to also take time to slow down and just get *–still!* And no, I am not talking about sitting still while watching television or when driving in your car because you are still preoccupied. What I mean is getting really still. Shutting out all of the distractions and in quiet solitude hearing the great voice inside of you, which helps to guide your path and daily steps. Yes, I am indeed suggesting that you should take some time each day to do absolutely nothing! This is a key factor in lowering your stress level, allowing you to recharge and become more productive!

Now, I know this is easier said than done. Believe me, I have been there. It may initially require you to intentionally schedule these breaks in your day, but just commit to giving it a try! Start by blocking out at least one period of "still time." You may need more depending on how fast your life moves.

During these interludes, try to unwind and appreciate things such as the beauty of nature and all that God has created. You could also use these moments to practice the art of breathing and meditation, clearing your head of clutter and refocusing your energy.

Getting still and silent is something that I've had to learn how to do, especially since I spend most of my day counseling or teaching. At home I have a dedicated space — a closet (which was emptied to remove all distractions) — that I go into each morning to meditate and pray. If I am not at home and having a particularly stressful day, I will go into the bathroom for a few moments of quiet.

With the lights off, I get still and wait to hear an inner whisper, which calms me so that I can successfully handle the tasks at hand.

In addition, realizing that nature settles my spirit and makes me slow down, I will often take a detour on the way home from work, go to a nearby park for a few minutes and enjoy the sounds, scents and sights of the outdoors. While sitting on a bench or taking a walk, I soak in the warmth of the sun, and experience ultimate peace. Alternatively, when possible I will take a trip to the beach where I enjoy the calming effects of the ocean waves. I am reassured in those serene moments that the same God who created such an amazing sea is also taking care of me.

If these ideas work for you, awesome! If you would prefer to retreat in another way, just remember to take the time to find a place to quiet the noise in your life so that you can get a greater sense of clarity. Take a moment now to reflect on these two questions: *How often do you take time out of your day to be still? What are some ways that you are willing to incorporate "stillness" into your busy day to reset and refocus?* Think about it, write it down, then start the process of getting still to hear your greatest voice.

Dr. Tiffany's Pearl of Wisdom:

Intentionally schedule still times until "stillness" becomes a habit.

Personal Reflections

(Take time to write down your thoughts on how you can get still and De-Stress for Success)

TIP 3: YOU GOTTA MOVE IT

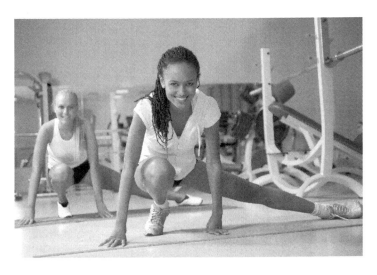

There's no substitute for exercising, so simply — move your body!

Let's talk about the power of exercise and why this is a key remedy for stress. When you are stressed, you already know that your brain releases hormones such as cortisol, norepinephrine and adrenaline. In addition, we have already established that in the short term, these hormones are good for you and enable you to complete tasks during the day; but when they are in your system for extended periods of time, they can actually backfire on you. Yes, the same hormones that are initially intended to help you complete tasks such as planning for that big wedding day, acing that test or getting through that important presentation or assignment at work, can actually hurt you if you are not careful. It is vital to find ways to redirect and lower these stress hormones so that they can be kept in check before they wreak havoc on your body.

When you exercise you are not only working to get into shape and improve your cardiovascular health, you are also releasing powerful anti-stress hormones better known as **endorphins**. They are our pleasure hormones that make us feel good, elevate our mood and act as agents to reverse the damaging effects of stress, anxiety and much more. In fact, endorphins are almost as potent as antidepressants and are a vital part of our body's defense mechanism to keep our lives in balance. With routine physical activity, endorphins are stimulated which actually stop the release of the stress hormones.

Now at this point you may be saying, *"I would love to exercise, but I just don't have the time."* I can definitely understand this concern. However, it is important to realize that in order for you to effectively take care of others, you have to first take care of yourself. If you are out of shape, either mentally or physically, how will you be able to maintain the stamina to perform at your best and make the great impact in this world that you are predestined for? That is why the busier you are, the more important it is to make physical activity an essential part of your daily routine.

Exercise is beneficial on many different levels, and when it comes to stress management, it is undeniably one of the greatest weapons that we possess.

Start small! Any steps taken to lead an active lifestyle will help. Look at your schedule and figure out where you can fit in at least 10 minutes a day. Most of us can do that, even if you commit to doing things such as avoiding the elevator, taking short walks at lunch time, dancing to a few of your favorite songs or running around as you play with your kids at the park (I often recommend this to my patients with small children as a great way to spend quality time with their little ones while getting in good exercise at the same time). Also, if you live or work in a facility with stairwells and long hallways, pledge to use those as intentional means of getting in a little exercise as you power walk to your destination rather than stroll. You will be surprised. Even these small bursts of physical activity can add up over the course of the day if you are consistent. Then diligently work your way up to the recommended

30-45 minutes of exercise a day most days of the week. As you do this, you will be amazed at how good you'll begin to feel, not to mention that you will have a sense of accomplishment, knowing that you have taken steps toward improving your overall health.

Dr. Tiffany's Pearl of Wisdom:

Make your workout fun by doing your favorite
activity such as walking, jogging, dancing, lifting
weights or jumping rope. One of the best times to
exercise is in the morning to kick-start your day.
But if you are going to exercise after work, do it
before you go home so that you don't allow life's
distractions to deter you from achieving your goals.

Use the log on the pages that follow to help track
how you are staying active and fit. But don't stop
there! Continue to track your exercise in an activity
journal or a health app, which will **keep you**
focused on your goals.

Here are a few suggestions for apps that I like to share with my patients:

MyFitnessPal and MyPlate Calorie Tracker™

Both of these free apps are available on your mobile device and allow you to track the calories that you consume as well as the amount of calories that you expend each day. They also help you to balance your meals by keeping you informed of the nutritional content of the food that you are eating.

The Johnson & Johnson Official 7 Minute Workout™

A great app that is ideal for those on the go! It also adjusts its level of difficulty based on your individual fitness level. There are additional workouts that are longer than 7 minutes in this app if you have more time, but on the days that you are busy, it will allow you to get structured exercise in a very short period of time.

Map My Fitness™

These developers have created multiple exercise apps including **Map My Walk™** and **Map My Run™** that use GPS features to view detailed statistics regarding your workout.

Fitbit™

A simple way to live healthier and more active. This app allows you to not only track your activity throughout the day, but also allows you to monitor other things such as food, sleep and weight.

C25K- 5K Trainer™

A practical app to get beginners who were previously couch potatoes to become 5K distance runners in only six to eight weeks.

Dr. Tiffany Lowe-Payne

Activity Log

(Write down your activity to help you keep track of how you are staying active and fit.)

Date	Activity	Length of Time
Ex. 1/12/16	**Zumba**	**30 min.**

*Please Note: Before initiating any type of exercise program, please check with your personal health care provider to ensure that you are healthy enough to do so.

<u>Activity Log</u>

(Continue tracking your activity to determine how you are staying active and fit.)

Date	Activity	Length of Time

*Please Note: Before initiating any type of exercise program, please check with your personal health care provider to ensure that you are healthy enough to do so.

TIP 4: EXPERIENCE THE POWER OF POSITIVITY

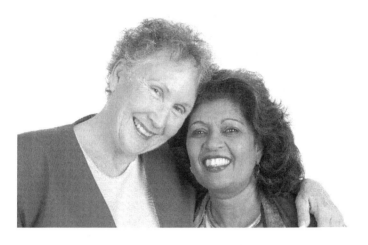

Positive thoughts in the beginning of your day help set the tone to keep the stress away.

Positive thinking will transform your life! I know this firsthand, having experienced the manifestations of a renewed mind through faith. But before I tell you my personal story, let me give you some of the scientific facts about the power of positivity. Similar to how your body reacts to physical activity or exercise, it is also influenced positively or negatively by the way you think and the words you profess. When you are a negative thinker or are under a lot of stress, it actually has an adverse impact on the function of your brain.

If you were to compare the brain of a person who is stressed and someone who is not, they are completely different. A person who feels over-whelmed has brain waves that are all over the place. On the other hand, if you look at the brain waves of someone who is reading, sitting still and generally in a relaxed state, their brain waves are very calm and settled. When someone is a negative thinker their mind is constantly stimulated and, as a result, their brain waves are in a chaotic state.

Disorderly brain waves trigger the over production of the cortisol hormone among others, which causes specific areas of the brain (i.e., the amygdala and hippocampus, the centers of emotion and memory) to become dysfunctional and ineffective. This can essentially make your mind begin to play tricks on you, causing you to become oversensitive to additional stimuli and perceive situations to be negative, even when they are not. As a result, you can develop irrational thoughts and fall victim to several conditions, including anxiety, paranoia, memory loss, impaired learning and sleep disturbance. In essence, negative thinking is actually toxic to your state of being!

On the other hand, when you are optimistic and incorporate affirmations into your daily life, positive thinking lowers your cortisol level and stimulates the release of good hormones such as serotonin and dopamine. Positivity lowers your stress levels and helps your brain to function at its highest capacity. Yes, consistently thinking positive, declaring words filled with joy and exposing yourself to encouraging stimuli (i.e., inspiring music or optimistic people) releases endorphins — just like exercise — and will ultimately support brain growth. As it grows, your brain will release more positive hormones, and your whole outlook on life can be transformed for the better. That is why positive thinking is so vital because it really does affect the quality of your health and how you feel. Once you master positive thinking, you will truly be able to renew your mind and manage stress in a way like never before.

I have personally experienced the power of positivity and also learned the importance of having the right people speak encouraging words into my life. This lesson came during one of the scariest and most shameful moments ever. When I was in my last year of college, I became pregnant. During this time, I was unmarried and my boyfriend and I had very little financial means. I was terrified! I also felt ashamed because this was not supposed to happen to me.

I grew up in the inner city of Camden, New Jersey, raised by a single mother of six children. According to society's low expectations and stereotypes of an "inner-city single mom" and her offspring, I was not supposed to become a physician. I must admit becoming a doctor was not an occupation that my peers and I were regularly exposed to at that time. My family did eventually move out of the city when I was a teen, but my mother continued to struggle and sacrifice to provide for our daily needs. The nicer things in life we had to go without. Needless to say, when I entered college and announced I was going to study to become a doctor, everyone was quite proud of me striving to become something that many had never imagined.

So, naturally I believed the news of me having a baby was going to be a huge disappointment. Not to mention that I was having sex out of wedlock, which would be definitely frowned upon by my family and support system, most of whom had deeply rooted religious beliefs. I was not supposed to be *"that girl!"* Instead I was going to be the one who would not be a statistic, rise above her circumstances and become a successful doctor! How could I ever do that now with a baby?

My boyfriend and I were so scared and regretful that initially we decided to have an abortion. We were just not ready to be parents. But ultimately, we decided to keep the baby and tell everyone the news. Indeed, there were some who said very hurtful things and tried to perpetuate the doubts that I already had in my mind. There were also those who questioned if my boyfriend would even stick around to care for our child. But, I thank God for the angels! Those who were placed in my life at the time to speak words of wisdom and hope. Those people who spread their wings and guided me along the way. Because of their love, I was able to shake the feelings of guilt and condemnation as I recognized that for whatever the reason, God had chosen me to be a vessel and a shepherd for this child. I had to learn not to be ashamed of the seed that He had placed in me to grow. Indeed, the child was not the sin. This new responsibility, in fact, strengthened my courage to pursue my dreams relentlessly. I was more motivated than ever to be successful because I was going to have a family to provide for.

Now, when I look back some twenty years later, I am truly blessed that I have had a successful medical career, my firstborn son is now a college student himself at a prestigious university and my college sweetheart never left my side. Despite what some people told me, we married and have enjoyed a life together as lovers and partners for the past 15 years. I am so thankful for those individuals who lifted me up, infused me with positive messages and never let me fall. These people taught me the importance of speaking *"life"* over my situations, even if there are others who doubt. Because of their influence of positivity, I am now able to use the platform that I have as a doctor and an overcomer to encourage you. **If you think well — and you do well — then you will indeed be well.** Now it's your turn!

1. *What changes would you like to see in your personal life or career?*

2. In what ways a*re you trying to improve your health?*

3. *Are you wanting to improve your marriage?*

4. *Are you looking to advance on your job or longing to venture out on your own as an entrepreneur?*

5. *Are you concerned about your loved ones?*

Begin to speak positive affirmations over what you are hoping for and work earnestly, having the faith to believe that it will come to pass and then let God do the rest! But as you wait in expectation, begin to praise Him in advance acknowledging that you have full confidence that He will supply all of your needs because He always has your back! Remember, as a man thinketh, so is he (Proverbs 23:7). So break the chains of negative thinking and begin to transform your life from the inside out!

Dr. Tiffany's Pearl of Wisdom:

Your ability to think positive influences the power that you have over stress and challenging situations. Train your brain to do a "hard stop" when negative thoughts arise. Refuse to allow doubt to dictate your life. You can do this by speaking the result that you desire, even before it is reality. Also, refine your inner circle and environment. Surround yourself with individuals and things that are inspiring, not draining. It is important to realize that faith by itself is not enough. In fact, "faith without works is dead" (James 2: 14-26, NIV). So be sure to work diligently as you wait in faithful anticipation and begin to watch the power of positivity work **wonders** in your life.

<u>Personal Reflections</u>

Use this space to reflect on the things that you desire. Then write positive affirmations over those things you identified, and witness the power of positivity in your life.

TIP 5: VALUE YOUR SLEEP

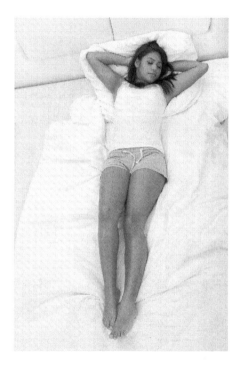

The notion that those who are most successful have to regularly "burn the midnight oil" is detrimental to your health and your business.

There are so many different reasons why getting a good night's sleep is important to our overall well-being, and I want to take time to discuss a few. Although it is a well-known fact that on average we need between six to eight hours of sleep a night, many people who have busy lifestyles will openly admit that they do not routinely meet this goal. Studies have also proven that women actually need 15-20 minutes more sleep each day than their male counterparts. Perhaps, this is due to the fact that as women, we spend the majority of our day multi-tasking. By the time we lie down to rest, our energy reserve at times is essentially depleted.

For as many advances that we have made in our careers — blazing trails, knocking down professional doors, and raising the roof on the glass ceiling — there are still many traditional roles in effect. We constantly juggle our roles as moms, daughters, sisters, caregivers, companions and friends. With the combination of these demands, we can overtask ourselves at the expense of our health if we do not take the time to get the proper rest.

It is extremely important to get a good night's sleep, as this is a vital part of ensuring that we are properly rejuvenated to handle our daily demands. Contrary to what some may believe, it is not just about the amount of sleep that we get, it's also about the quality. If you regularly deprive yourself of good quality rest, every aspect of your body and your health will be impacted making you vulnerable to sickness and disease. Inadequate sleep will make you less efficient and will cause you to be virtually incapable of successfully managing your responsibilities.

As discussed earlier in the book, cortisol is a powerful and potentially detrimental hormone that will once again rear its ugly head when you are sleep deprived. If your sleep cycle is disrupted and you deny your body of rest, your circadian rhythm (internal biological clock that is synchronized to light-dark cycles) will be thrown off, your cortisol levels will elevate as your tired body experiences extreme stress and your regenerative system will begin to shut down. Sounds serious, huh? That's because it is, and your body will let you know when you have cheated yourself of good sleep as you begin to have various symptoms including increased irritability, anger management issues and feelings of anxiety. In fact, lack of quality sleep has been linked to several ailments such as obesity, chronic fatigue syndrome, depression, memory loss and, in severe cases, heart disease and stroke. So, no matter how busy you are, make good sleep a priority at the end of the day! Your body will thank you.

So, what are some ways to ensure that you get quality sleep?

You must initially determine that you do not have a medical condition that is hindering you from getting the rest that you need. Medical conditions such as sleep apnea that cause you to have pauses in breathing when you are sleep, chronic pain, asthma or even mental health issues including depression and anxiety can significantly impact your ability to have a restful night. In these instances, addressing and controlling the underlying condition can actually be the best course of action and ultimately lead to a cure.

After a medical condition is ruled out by a

professional, you could consider trying medication sleep aides to see if they help you get a good night's sleep. However, there are also practical techniques you can add to your nightly routine that will help you naturally prepare for peaceful slumber.

First, try to limit the length of time that you take naps during the day to 20 minutes or less. Anything longer than that can impair your ability to get good sleep at night. Additionally, it is important to remove all unnecessary stimuli. Your bedroom should be your sanctuary, a place where you can go at the end of the day to unwind, relax and rejuvenate. Create a calming atmosphere with delightful fragrances, comfy bedding and even soft music. Relaxation techniques such as light reading, yoga, meditation or prayer have been shown to be excellent ways to relieve stress so that you can have peaceful rest. Furthermore, try to avoid things that are stimulating right before bedtime such as vigorous exercise, alcohol, caffeine or intense conversations with others. These activities will actually hinder you from lulling off into a deep sleep where the bulk of your rejuvenation occurs.

You also want to be careful about watching unnerving programs on television, including suspenseful thrillers or horror movies, which will actually stimulate your senses.

Finally, one of the biggest stimulants in our lives and potentially one of the greatest things that robs us of our sleep is our dependence on, and in some cases addiction to, technology. Yes, the fact that you have your cell phone and other gadgets right next to you when you go to bed could easily be considered as **public enemy No. 1** against getting the sleep that your body is craving! I will talk more about this in the next tip.

Now I cannot forget about those who have alternative schedules and may work at night or on split shifts. You are among a special group of individuals who find that it is virtually impossible feel fully rested as you are trying to sleep during a period of time when the majority of the world is awake and active. This is a medical condition known as "shift work disorder." Trying to sleep during the day is an adjustment, as our natural circadian rhythm is wired for us to sleep at night when it is dark; so getting deep sleep during the day requires you to be more creative. While applying many of the techniques mentioned earlier can help you to successfully drift off to sleep, also try the following: Get room darkening window coverings to create the feeling of night and help to keep your room cool; find a place in the house where there will be the least amount of interruptions from others who are awake or use ear plugs to block out noise; and, turn off the ringer and vibration on your phone.

Dr. Tiffany's Pearl of Wisdom:

Getting proper sleep is essential. Remember it is not about quantity but rather the quality of sleep that you get. Make your room a sanctuary that you come home to at the end of a long day. Then settle your brain, lie your head down and drift away into a deep and peaceful sleep.

Personal Reflections

Think about your room. What are some things that may be stopping you from getting a good night's sleep? Use this space to reflect on what changes you can make to remove those distractions so that you can sleep in peace?

TIP 6: GET RID OF THE GADGETS

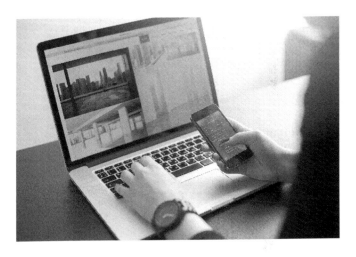

You don't have to always respond to everything right away.

There is no doubt that in this Digital Age, technology has made some things in our lives more accessible and more convenient. For instance, we can enjoy all kinds of information at our fingertips on our many devices. But what is meant to be good for us can become detrimental if we do not put limits on its consumption. Seriously, think about how often you are looking at some form of technology throughout the day. Consider how frequently you sleep with your cell phone right next to your bed. Having cell phones close to our beds can affect our sleep even when we have them on vibrate. Admit it, we have all become conditioned to hearing those tiny vibrations without the ringer, which in turn can and will disrupt your sleep during the night. In addition, even the light emitting off of your mobile screen can impact your sleep by fooling your mind and body to think that it is daytime when it's not. Practice turning off your phone completely or putting it someplace away from the bed where you cannot easily reach for it out of sheer habit.

Yes, get rid of the gadgets — the cell phones, computers, tablets, etc. — at least for a portion of the day and at night, and watch some of your stress disappear.

Now if I am being transparent then I must confess that before I could talk to other people about this topic, I had to examine myself first because I too was once hooked on my gadgets. Let's face it, our devices make it extremely easy to gather information so that we can stay in the loop about current events and be connected to friends and family. However, because of my former preoccupation with my cell phone and iPad, I often found myself stressing about things that were essentially out of my control. It also caused me to procrastinate and be less productive. Before I knew it, a few minutes of catch-up would easily turn into an hour or more. Once I learned how to put limits on the time that I spent surfing the internet or catching up on social media, I began to feel my mind settle, which ultimately helped me to refocus my priorities. I realized how much time I was wasting on things that weren't very important.

There is a time and place for your gadgets, and there is a time when you should put them down. My suggestions for implementing this healthy habit include creating a morning routine that does not involve looking at your cell phone for at least 30 minutes after you awake. In addition, turn off notifications after a certain hour or when you are resting. Also, try scheduling times throughout the day when you will look at email or connect with others via your devices.

Remember, you can have too much of a good thing. Don't let technology become lord over you!

Dr. Tiffany's Pearl of Wisdom:

Take a moment to think about it. Over the next few days, track how much time you spend looking at some form of technology. Then honestly answer the following questions:

1. Does the amount of time that you spend with your gadgets affect your productivity?
2. Do your gadgets affect your ability to relax?
3. Are they robbing you of the opportunity to spend uninterrupted quality time with your loved ones?

If you've answered yes to any of these questions, try placing limits on the use of your gadgets. Create a "technology-free time zone," where you'll be able to focus and complete tasks more efficiently. You could also enjoy spending precious moments with your family and friends or participate in an activity that brings you happiness and a **sense of peace.**

Personal Reflections

Write out your plan to schedule technology-free times in your day. Then enjoy the benefits as the stress melts away.

TIP 7: MASTER THE ART OF SAYING "NO"

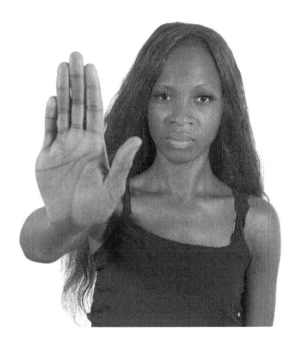

Your need to please everyone can actually backfire on you and be a primary source for your downfall.

Saying *"No"* goes hand-in-hand with being keenly aware of your limits. Know when you have reached your max, then practice the art of saying, *"No."* This is probably one of the most important tips because if we can learn when and where to use this word, then we will never feel like we are stretched too thin and overextended again! It is such an easy word, but for many it's one of the hardest to say. It is hard because we naturally want to please and help people. We want everyone to like us and we want people (especially our bosses and those we love) to believe that we can do it all. The problem is that when we continually say *"Yes"* or *"Sure"* and allow others to add more responsibilities to our plate, we will eventually burn out. Learning *how* to say *"No"* and knowing *when* to say it is crucial in lowering our stress levels. It is also really good for our personal brands. No one wants to be in a position where they cannot live up to expectations by biting off more than they can chew. People will actually learn to respect you more if you are aware of your personal limits and decline when you are feeling overloaded instead of saying *"Yes"* and doing a less than optimal job. Saying *"No"* at times will certainly save you from the unwanted consequences of over-promising and under-delivering.

An important part of mastering how to say *"No"* also means denying yourself at times. This is vital because the decisions that we make in an impulsive manner can ultimately backfire on us if we are not careful. Practice saying *"No"* to things that you know are not good for you — like that extra piece of chocolate cake when you are trying to eat healthier; procrastinating on that major assignment when the deadline is quickly approaching; or even learning how not to react to everything—including, at times, your own feelings. In instances such as these, you have to choose to resist going down a doomed path of feeling guilty, stressed or anxious as a result of your decision. It does require understanding which battles to fight and when it is best to stay silent or wave the proverbial white flag for the sake of maintaining the peace. Again this can be difficult to do, especially when you may feel that your point of view is the correct one. However, if you are someone who has to constantly prove a point, you are going to be an extremely stressed person. So when you are faced with the option of whether it is worth using the time and energy to defend your position on a potentially heated topic, ask yourself this one question: ***Will the point you want to make significantly impact the quality of your life if you are not heard?*** If the answer is no, then you may want to exercise your right to remain silent and let it go!

Dr. Tiffany's Pearl of Wisdom:

Know your limits. Learn the art of saying "No."
When you do, you will find that it is quite freeing.
When you say "No" let it go and worry no more!
There are many ways to say "No", such as "It's
not my season for this," "The energy isn't aligned,"
or just plain "No, not at this time." However you
decide to deliver the message, find strength and
freedom in refusing to get involved in things that
will stress you out or stretch you too thin.

Personal Reflections

Take time to write down all of your commitments. This
should include obligations in both your personal and
professional life.

Personal Reflections

Now thoroughly consider each commitment. Which of them is helping you to flourish and which is actually causing you to perish. Once you determine this, begin to remove the things that are draining you out of your life.

TIP 8: UNLOCK THE POWER OF PRAYER

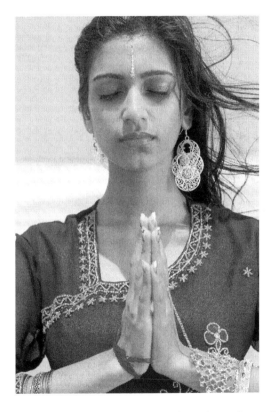

The quality of our health is directly tied to our ability to have faith.

Several studies show that a person's overall quality of health, especially in dealing with difficult situations, is directly affected by his or her level of faith. In addition, engaging in practices such as regular prayer and meditation have been shown to increase your levels of the "happy hormones," serotonin and dopamine, and lower your stress hormones, cortisol and noradrenaline. There is also evidence that the mortality rate is 37 percent lower in individuals who possess a strong belief system and that they handle stressors much better than those who do not. For many, this is not a huge surprise.

Here is the catch! While many individuals profess that they are faith-filled and believe there is a higher presence that acts as their healer, sustainer and protector, in times of great storm they forget to utilize the power source within them. Over the years, individuals have built up their faith, attending worship services and reading scriptures about people who have overcome when they have activated their faith, and yet they fail to use their own when needed.

If I am being completely honest, I too have been guilty of this in the past. But what I have learned is that if we take our concerns to the one who we believe holds our density in His hands, then our faith becomes a source of comfort and will lower our stress.

As a Christian, I truly believe the Bible when it says that we "should not be anxious or fearful for anything; if we make our requests known, God will give us a peace that surpasses all understanding (Philippians 4:6-7)." The Word also says "we can do all things through Him which gives us strength (Philippians. 4:13)" and "He knows the plans that have already been laid out for us (Jeremiah 29:11)." "He already knew our end before our beginning (Isaiah 46:10)."

Whatever doctrine you choose to believe, if you are a person of faith remember to first confide in the source that drives your existence before you seek the advice of anyone else. Make time to regularly pray, meditate, fast and refocus yourself as you strengthen your faith. Now, you may ask what's the difference between prayer and meditation? Great question, as it is important to understand the difference between the two. Prayer is the time we spend with God, letting Him know all of our fears, concerns and desires. This is an active time of communication where we can discuss our issues and seek to find the answers that we need. On the other hand, as mentioned earlier in Tip 2, meditation is our ability to sit still and listen while patiently waiting to hear from God so that He can give us the answers to our questions and order our daily steps. It is vital to make time for both prayer and meditation as we develop our relationship with God, to ensure we are truly hearing His voice before we make decisions that could affect the rest of our lives.

At this point, it is also important to mention another big cause of stress in the lives of many. It is the overwhelming burden that comes along with the spirit of "unforgiveness" (the inability to forgive when something bad happens to you). This is not only a spiritual principle, as scriptures frequently encourage us to forgive *(see Matthew 10:8, Luke*

6:27-28 and John 15:12) but it is also validated in scientific studies as well. Similar to negative thinking, unforgiveness has been shown to be poisonous, affecting the normal function of your brain as it causes the release of stress hormones, decreasing your immune system and making you susceptible to a host of illnesses. These illnesses include extreme anger and bitterness, anxiety, depression and eating disorders, which can all be debilitating, as well as high blood pressure and heart disease. In fact, studies have shown that unforgiveness is just as much of a risk factor for heart disease as smoking, because they both produce an inflammatory response and place extraordinary stressors on the normal function of your heart.

Take a moment to think about this. *Have you been deeply hurt by someone? Have you experienced a tragic event in your life and need help to move beyond your past? Do you harbor feelings of unforgiveness or resentment in your heart?* If you have been hurt, either mentally or physically and feel bound by the chains of unforgiveness,

I encourage you to start the process of complete healing by first learning to forgive. This does not mean that you have to condone wrong actions, nor does it imply that you have to allow yourself to be hurt again. But what it does symbolize is that by understanding your value, you are willing to make a conscious decision not to allow the spirit of unforgiveness and its toxic effects to destroy you. Just as a diamond endures a great deal of pressure before it reveals it true luster, you too can overcome the burdens of your past by learning to forgive so that you can heal, restore your joy and begin to shine. I know learning to forgive may be very difficult for some, but with the help of professionals such as your doctor, therapist or minister and the power of prayer and meditation, it can be done.

"Glass shatters but diamonds never break! You are a diamond, never let anyone or anything dull your luster."~ Dr. Tiffany

I am a personal witness to the power of prayer and meditation. I can remember a very stressful moment in my life and career when I found myself right in the center of a crisis. I was told by my employer that the medical practice I was happy to have, the one that I helped to build and had invested so much time and energy in was going to close. Despite all of the education that I had, all of my years of experience as a physician and all of the effort spent building that practice, it was over and there was nothing I could do to save it. I was blindsided.

Now, I could have allowed this to take me down the path of despair, but because of my strong faith I was able to quickly remind myself that the God who I love had the power to take what seemed hopeless and give it new life. As a result, I did the only thing that I knew to do during that time, which was pray! I began to speak the promises of the scriptures that dwelled in my heart and asked for clarity of why this was happening. That's when I was given a breakthrough revelation: God needed me to shift to another level to incite transformation in the lives of

His people! I am a doctor with a heart for people and as much as I loved to encourage and inspire my patients in the privacy of the examination room, He did not want me to get comfortable and limit my gifts to the four walls of that office. In fact, He needed me to use that same voice to go out into the world and seek to empower many, helping those who are broken become whole. He also reminded me that the happiness I felt was a superficial feeling that could easily be taken away, and that true joy comes from within. I didn't want to just be happy. I wanted joy.

Furthermore, God helped me to realize that the changes that were about to occur in my career weren't even about me; it was greater than me. It was actually about you as you're hopefully being empowered and blessed by reading this book. This next season in my life was going to be about all of the people that I would help understand that healthy living is more than a physical principle. It's also a spiritual expectation that starts with the renewal of our minds (Romans 2:12), so that we can live healthy and whole. So trust me, prayer works! Try it for yourself and watch the manifestations of God's purpose for you come alive and help you to live in perfect peace (Isaiah 26:3).

To manage stress even during the most trying situations, pray. Give God your best! Begin a routine that allows you to spend time with Him first thing in the morning when you feel the most rejuvenated. Then continue to meditate and communicate with Him throughout the day. Read an encouraging word or worship with Him through song. Write out the things that are stressing you in a letter so that you can clearly know what to ask for in prayer. Make God your first point of contact when you need help and believe that He will give you exactly what you need.

In addition, don't be afraid to speak with your physician(s) about your faith and let them know that you want it to be an important part of your health care plan. Studies have shown that while over 90 percent of Americans believe in a higher being and 77 percent of them want it included as a part of their medical care, only 10-20 percent of physicians actually address their patients' spirituality and incorporate it into their treatment plans.

That is why I love being an osteopathic physician! Spirituality is deeply rooted in our principles and reflected in the many quotes by Andrew Taylor Still, founder of the first American school of osteopathic medicine in 1892, who said, *"God is the father of osteopathy, and I am not ashamed of the child of his mind."* A.T. Still truly believed in the importance of a holistic approach to medicine. In fact, the first tenet of osteopathic medicine requires that we, as osteopathic physicians, understand that the body is an integrated unit of mind, body and spirit. We cannot separate any aspect of this principle if we are looking to treat the whole patient. This is also a belief system that many authorities in healthcare are now adopting. In 1998, the World Health Organization (WHO) modified the preamble to its constitution to state that, *"Health is a dynamic state of complete physical, mental, spiritual and social well-being and not merely the absence of disease or infirmity."*

Prayer works indeed! Try it and see that you will not only feel better, but you will have a clearer perspective over your life that will place you on the road to success.

Dr. Tiffany's Pearl of Wisdom:

Prayer and meditation, along with the ability to think positive and to forgive, are essential to lowering your stress. Prayer is your direct line to talk to and hear from God, so that you can receive the answers that you'll need to handle every situation in your life. If this is not a regular part of your daily routine, I challenge you to give it a try. Make a commitment to yourself that you will set aside some time to go to a quiet place, pray and meditate each day. See for yourself that prayer really does work!

Personal Reflections

What issues in your life may be causing you stress and negatively affecting the way you feel? Write out your specific concerns, then use this as a guide to help you know how to pray and ask God for guidance.

Here are some scriptures that I love, which you can reflect on and use as promises when you are praying to God about your health (according to the King James Version of the Bible):

1. *"Beloved I wish above all things that thou mayest prosper and be in health, even as thy soul prospereth."* (3 John 1:2)

2. *"A merry (cheerful) heart doeth good like a medicine: but a broken spirit drieth the bones."* (Proverbs 17:22)

3. *"Behold, I will bring health and cure, and I will cure them, and will reveal unto them the abundance of peace and truth."* (Jeremiah 33:6)

4. *"Pleasant words are as an honeycomb, sweet to the soul and health to the bones."* (Proverbs 16:24)

5. *"My son (daughter), attend (listen) to my words; incline thine ear unto my sayings. Let them not depart from thine eyes; keep them in the midst of thine heart; for they are life unto those who find them and health to all their flesh (the entire body)."* (Proverbs 4:20-22)

6. *"Do not be wise in thine own eyes; fear the Lord and depart from evil. It shall be health to thy navel (body) and marrow (nourishment) to thy bones."* (Proverbs 3:7-8)

7. *"What? Know ye not (don't you know) that your body is the temple of the Holy Ghost which is in you, which ye have (received) of God? and ye are not your own; For ye are bought with a price. Therefore, glorify (honor) God in your body and in your spirit, which are God's."* (1 Corinthians 6:19-20)

8. *"Be careful (do not be anxious) for nothing, but in everything by prayer and supplication with thanksgiving let your request be made known to God. And the peace which of God which passeth all understanding, shall keep your hearts and minds through Christ Jesus."* (Philippians 4:6-7)

9. *"Death and life are in the power of the tongue, and they that love it shall eat the fruit thereof."* (Proverbs 18:21)

10. *"But he was wounded for our transgressions, he was bruised for our iniquities; the chastisement of our peace was upon him; and with his stripes we are healed."* (Isaiah 53:5)

TIP 9: IMPROVE YOUR WORK-LIFE BALANCE

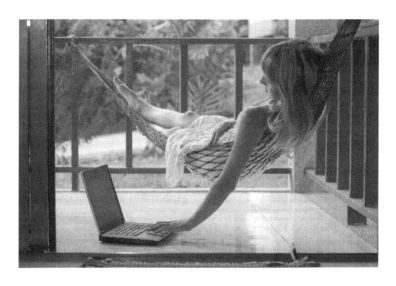

You're no good to anyone else,
until you are first good to yourself.

If you are a workaholic, this tip is just for you! One of the greatest stressors that people have in their lives is their jobs. Work-related stress, which is so common and said to be the biggest cause of **"burnout syndrome,"** is one of the primary issues that drives patients to their doctors. If this sounds familiar to you, it is important to develop a sense of balance and learn how to put the work down. This is especially true for entrepreneurs and "solo-preneurs," who work from home and lose track of time because they do not have to leave the premises. Make a pledge to yourself to set realistic limits on the amount of time that you spend on work each day and then schedule time for yourself to begin to reclaim the whole you!

If you have concerns that you may not be able to get everything done or the thought of committing to a "quitting time" raises your stress meter, here are a few things that will help you to stay on track. First, figure out the time of day when your mind is the clearest and you can perform at your best. This will vary for everyone as some people are naturally more efficient during the morning while others work better as night owls. Once you identify when you work best, consider these your *"hours of power,"* the time that you are the most efficient and the most creative. Try to do as much as you can during this time. You will not only be more productive and get the maximum return on your labor and investment, but you will also begin to feel your level of stress decrease as you enjoy the satisfaction of completing tasks.

In addition, use your resources wisely. Take the same gadgets that you rely on for information and use them to help you get better organized. Although we, as a connected society, depend on gadgets, most people do not take advantage of all of the features "smart technology" has to offer. Optimize your tools. When used correctly, they can be the key to becoming more efficient and *"de-stressed."* Finally, learn how to ask for help! Avoid the mindset that if you want something done right, you have to do it all yourself. Otherwise known as the *"super-hero"* mentality, when you are convinced that you are the only person who can get the job done. Learn to delegate. It will not only lessen your load, but it will also help to develop and cultivate the gifts of others around you. This will benefit everyone.

Dr. Tiffany's Pearl of Wisdom:

I challenge you to spend the next seven days tracking the times of day when you perform at your optimal level. Then adjust your schedule and plan to do your most important work during those times. Afterward implement 30 minutes of exercise, time to connect with loved ones and quiet moments for you (I'll talk more about this in the next tip). Schedule times where you are still and can hear from God and plan your six to eight hours of sleep. Doing these things regularly will improve *your* work-life balance.

Here are some suggestions for free mobile apps to help you get better organized, more efficient and less stressed:

Hours Keeper™ helps to keep track of your hours worked. Also generates invoices and calculates your earnings.

Super Notes™ allows you to store notes, record lectures and presentations, compile to-do-lists and much more.

Wunderlist™ helps you create to-do-lists and notifies you with reminders to complete tasks or meet your deadlines.

Speak and Translate™ is a voice and text translator that allows you to effectively communicate with your peers in other countries in several languages.

TIP 10: ENJOY "ME TIME"

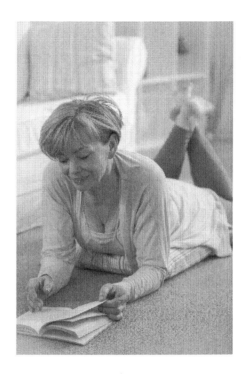

You are your greatest asset.
Take care of your personal needs first.

You have to have *"me" time*! At the end of the day, after you have done everything for everybody else, find the time to take care of you. Actually, this should not be the last thing you do, but indeed it should be one of the first. Remind yourself that the better you take care of yourself, the better you will be able to care for others. This is not something that is easy for people to do, and it is especially not easy for women because as nurturers we can easily put the needs of others in front of our own. You have to pamper yourself intentionally!

Pampering yourself does not have to always take the whole day, although that would be great! When I speak at conferences, workshops and even one-on-one with my patients, I usually recommend that people start with just an hour a day. For 30 minutes, do some kind of physical activity (for the reasons that we discussed earlier). For the other 30 minutes, do something relaxing for yourself. This does not have to be expensive. It can be as simple as taking a soothing bath, taking a leisurely walk or reading a novel. And if you are able, get a massage, head to the beauty salon or even take a trip every once in a while. The point is that every day we should be doing something for ourselves to refocus and rejuvenate. As you do this, you will feel yourself become completely restored. This will allow you to live and perform at your best — and that is the goal, total health and wellness from the inside out!

I would be remiss if I did not include the importance of intimacy with the person you love. This is most definitely an effective way to take time for yourself that is not only fun, strengthens your relationship and provides personal satisfaction, it has also been scientifically proven to immediately lower your stress levels. In healthy relationships, intimacy is vital for your physical and mental health. Now, a little cuddle time is always good, but let's take it even one step further. Yes, I am talking about the benefits of sex! This may be an uncomfortable subject for some people to consider as a means for stress relief, but I want you to consider this. When you engage in sexual activity, your heart rate naturally increases and depending on how vigorous your session is and how creative you are during foreplay, you can burn 100 to 300 calories per hour, if not more. In addition, as you perform thrusts, you are actually using pelvic and stomach muscles, which when worked become stronger and helps to improve bladder control and strengthens your core. For many, that beats a session at the gym any day! In addition, as you reach your climax your body releases hormones – endorphins and prolactin, which helps to relax and lull you into a deep sleep. Unlike our male counterparts, women have the ability to have multiple orgasms, which means each time you reach a climax, your stress level continues to lessen and your feelings of relaxation increase.

However you decide to escape, just remember to take time for yourself. Your mind and body will thank you!

Dr. Tiffany's Pearl of Wisdom:

Take a moment to reflect. Do you intentionally schedule regular times to pamper yourself? If so, what are some ways? If not, what can you reasonably add into your life to begin to take time for you? Remember to have "me-time," relax, rejuvenate and enjoy the benefits of taking time for the most important person in your life — **you!**

In Conclusion...

The principles mentioned in this book do not only represent the physical manifestations of stress on your health, but also speaks to the quality of your mental and spiritual health as well. As a faith-filled physician who is committed to helping women who are broken become whole, I truly believe that healthy living starts on the inside before it can manifest outside. It is imperative that you renew your mindset to restore your body, replenish your spirit and strengthen your inner woman. So if the chronic stressors in your life are starting to affect your health, I recommend that you begin to think about how you can change your lifestyle and your thought process to better manage your stress. I challenge you to consider adopting the techniques mentioned in this book and make them a consistent part of your daily routine. **Then after 90 days, I encourage you to retake the stress test** assessment test in Tip 1 to see if your score improves. I am confident that if you do, you will not only recognize that you are transforming for the better, but you will be happy that your stress levels will be much lower, you will be more focused and ultimately more successful in every aspect of your life!

A few final words ...

As you apply this book's tips to your life, do it in ways that work best for you by implementing them into things that you already enjoy doing. Start simple and make it fun. Do not try to live in perfection as that brings a separate stressor all of its own. Instead just strive to walk in excellence as you make healthy changes to your life. Keep in mind that some of these changes may take time for you to master; I know that was the case for me. However, once you decide that you want to experience real change and take action with intentional steps, you will be able to break the cycle of negative habits and begin to **De-Stress for Success!**

Finally, make sure that you have a primary care doctor and that you are getting physicals on a regular basis to constantly evaluate your overall health. Annual exams are an opportunity to know your numbers (cholesterol, blood sugar, blood pressure are the big three), and to ensure that you are up to date with preventive screening tests that will keep your body healthy.

It is time to start your journey to living healthy and whole. I have faith that you can achieve this, and please know that I'm here for you as an advocate to help you make the rest of your life, the best of your life!

Share your thoughts about this book with Dr. Tiffany! Visit her page on Amazon or **DrTiffanyLowePayne.com** where you can submit a review.

Also visit her website and sign up to stay connected as you learn more about **The Institute of Transformational Health & Wellness, Inc.,** and continue to receive great health tips, share your comments, ask health related questions, or inquire to **book Dr. Tiffany to speak at your next conference or event.**

References

Introduction

1. American Psychological Association, "Stress In America: Paying With Our Health," https://www.apa.org/news/press/releases/stress/2014/stress-report.pdf (February 4, 2015)

2. American Psychological Association, "Stress Effects on the Body," http://www.apa.org/helpcenter/stress-body.aspx

3. Mayo Clinic, "Chronic Stress Puts Your Health At Risk," http://www.mayoclinic.org/healthy-lifestyle/stress-management/in-depth/stress/art-20046037 (July 11, 2013)

4. Psychology Today, "Are You Stressed Out? Take The Quiz," https://www.psychologytoday.com/blog/just-listen/201010/are-you-stressed-out-take-the-quiz (October 9, 2010)

5. Selye, Hans MD, PhD, D. Sc, F.R.S.C., "Stress and The General Adaptation Syndrome," The British Medical Journal, June 17, 1950.

Tip 1: Identify the Problem: "The Stress Test"

1. American Psychological Association, "Stress In America: Paying With Our Health," https://www.apa.org/news/press/releases/stress/2014/stress-report.pdf (February 4, 2015)

2. American Psychological Association, "Stress Effects on the

Body," http://www.apa.org/helpcenter/stress-body.aspx

3. Mayo Clinic, "Chronic Stress Puts Your Health At Risk," http://www.mayoclinic.org/healthy-lifestyle/stress-management/in-depth/stress/art-20046037 (July 11, 2013)

Tip 2: Be Still

1. Colbert, Don DR. 2007 *The Seven Pillars of Health: The Natural Way To Better Health For Life*. Lake Mary, Florida: Siloam

2. King, Dana E. DR. 2000 *Faith, Spirituality and Medicine: Toward the Making of the Healing Practitioner*. Binghamton, NY: The Hawthorne Pastoral Press

Tip 3: You Gotta Move It

1. American Psychological Association, "Exercise Fuels The Brain's Stress Buffers," http://www.apa.org/helpcenter/exercise-stress.aspx

2. Anxiety and Depression Association of America, "Exercise For Stress and Anxiety," http://www.adaa.org/living-with-anxiety/managing-anxiety/exercise-stress-and-anxiety

3. Colbert, Don DR. 2007 *The Seven Pillars of Health: The Natural Way To Better Health For Life*. Lake Mary, Florida: Siloam

4. Harvard Health Publications, "Exercising To Relax," http://

www.health.harvard.edu/staying-healthy/exercising-to-relax Feb 1, 2011.

Tip 4: Experience the Power of Positivity

1. American Psychological Association, "Updating Positive and Negative Stimuli in Working Memory in Depression http://www.apa.org/pubs/journals/features/xge-139-4-654.pdf (2010)

2. Colbert, Don DR. 2007 *The Seven Pillars of Health: The Natural Way To Better Health For Life*. Lake Mary, Florida: Siloam

3. Johns Hopkins Medicine, "The Power of Positive Thinking," http://www.hopkinsmedicine.org/health/healthy_aging/healthy_mind/the-power-of-positive-thinking

4. King, Dana E. DR. 2000 *Faith, Spirituality and Medicine: Toward the Making of the Healing Practitioner*. Binghamton, NY: The Hawthorne Pastoral Press

5. Psychology Today, "Alpha Brain Waves Boost Creativity and Reduce Depression," https://www.psychologytoday.com/blog/the-athletes-way/201504/alpha-brain-waves-boost-cre-ativity-and-reduce-depression (April 17, 2015).

6. Psychology Today, " Happy Brain, Happy Life," https://www.psychologytoday.com/blog/prime-your-gray-cells/201108/happy-brain-happy-life (Aug 2, 2011).

7. Scott Coffey, PhD., Anne Banducci, PhD., Christine Vinci, PhD. "Common Questions About Cognitive Behavior Therapy For Psychiatric Disorders," *American Family Physician* Nov 1, 2015; 92(9) 807-812.

8. University of Minnesota, "How Do Thoughts and Emotions Impact Health," http://www.takingcharge.csh.umn.edu/enhance-your-wellbeing/health/thoughts-emotions/how-do-thoughts-emotions-impact-health

Tip 5: Value Your Sleep

American Psychological Association, "Stress and Sleep," http://www.apa.org/news/press/releases/stress/2013/sleep.aspx

Colbert, Don DR. 2007 *The Seven Pillars of Health: The Natural Way To Better Health For Life*. Lake Mary, Florida: Siloam

Harvard Medical School, "Consequences of Insufficient Sleep," http://healthysleep.med.harvard.edu/healthy/matters/consequences

National Sleep Foundation, "How Much Sleep Do We Really Need," https://sleepfoundation.org/how-sleep-works/how-much-sleep-do-we-really-need

National Sleep Foundation, "Shift Work Disorder," https://sleepfoundation.org/shift-work/content/non-medical-treatments-shift-work-disorder

National Sleep Foundation, "Sleep Disorders Problems,"
https://sleepfoundation.org/sleep-disorders-problems

Tip 6: Get Rid of The Gadgets
"The Dangers of Junk Sleep," http://www.cnn.com/
2014/06/12/health/junk-sleep-live-longer/index.html

Tip 7: Master The Art of Saying "No"
"Stress Relief: When and How to Say No," http://www.may-
oclinic.org/healthy-lifestyle/stress-management/in-depth/
stress-relief/art-20044494

Tip 8: Unlock the Power of Prayer
1. Aaron Saguil, MD, M.P.H., Karen Phelps, M.D., "The Spiritual Assessment", *American Family Physician* September 15,
2012 86(6): 546-550.
2. American Osteopathic Association, "Tenets of Osteopathic
Medicine," http://www.osteopathic.org/inside-aoa/about/lead-
ership/Pages/tenets-of-osteopathic-medicine.aspx
3. A.T. Still University, "Andrew Taylor Still: The Founder of
Osteopathic Medicine" http://www.atsu.edu/museum/ats/
4. "Blaming Others Can Ruin Your Health," http://www.cnn.-
com/2011/HEALTH/08/17/bitter.resentful.ep/
5. Christina M. Puchalski, M.D., MS, "The Role of Spirituality

in Health Care," *Baylor University Medical Center Proceedings* October 2001; 14(4): 352-357

6. Colbert, Don DR. 2007 *The Seven Pillars of Health: The Natural Way To Better Health For Life*. Lake Mary, Florida: Siloam

7. "Forgiveness, Your Health Depends On It," http://www.hopkinsmedicine.org/health/healthy_aging/healthy_connections/forgiveness-your-health-depends-on-it

8. Gowri Anandarajah, M.D., Ellen Hight, M.D., M.P.H., "Spirituality and Medical Practice: Using the HOPE Questions as a Practical Tool for Spiritual Assessment," *American Family Physician* January 1, 2001 1:63(1): 81-89

9. King, Dana E. DR. 2000 *Faith, Spirituality and Medicine: Toward the Making of the Healing Practitioner*. Binghamton, NY: The Hawthorne Pastoral Press

10. M. H. Kayat, "Spirituality in The Definition of Health: The World Health Organization's Point of View," http://www.medizin-ethik.ch/publik/spirituality_definition_health.htm

11. Up To Date, "Overview of Spirituality in Palliative Care," http://www.uptodate.com/contents/overview-of-spirituality-in-palliative-care (Updated October 7 2014).

Tip 9: Improve Your Work-life Balance

Allen, David. 2001 *Getting Things Done: The Art of Stress-Free Productivity*. New York, NY: Penguin Group

Mental Health America, " Work-Life Balance," http://www.-mentalhealthamerica.net/work-life-balance

Tip 10: Enjoy "Me-Time"

Amanda Gardner, " Ways Sex Affects Your Brain," http://abcnews.go.com/Health/ways-sex-affects-brain/story?id=28872676 (February 11, 2015)

Colbert, Don DR. 2007 *The Seven Pillars of Health: The Natural Way To Better Health For Life*. Lake Mary, Florida: Siloam

Health, "Pamper Yourself: 8 Natural Stress Relievers," http://www.health.com/health/gallery/0,,20794075,00.html

ABOUT THE AUTHOR
Meet Your Transformation and Rejuvenation
Expert, Dr. Tiffany Lowe-Payne

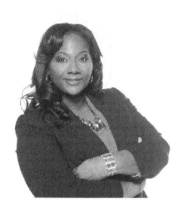

"Are you ready to be trans-formed? Decide today, to make the rest of your life, the best of your life!"
~Dr. Tiffany

Dr. Tiffany Lowe-Payne (Dr. Tiffany) is a highly respected, board-certified family physician and the founder/CEO of the **Institute of Transformational Health and Wellness, Inc.™** She is also an assistant professor of medicine, national speaker, author and media health expert on various issues seen in primary care. Whether she is treating patients in her office or appearing as a keynote speaker with her lighthearted and engaging personality, Dr. Tiffany is passionate about educating others on how to live healthy and whole.

Her goal is to transform lives from the inside out. Because of this, it is no wonder that she is affectionately known as **"A Doctor with a Heart for People™."** Her mission: *To help those who are broken become whole™* . She does this by combining her more than 15 years of experience as an osteopathic medical physician with her faith-filled principles to help individuals master the keys needed to live at their best — mind, body and spirit. She is your

Transformation and Rejuvenation Expert.™

Dr. Tiffany earned her Doctorate of Medicine degree from the University of Medicine and Dentistry of New Jersey School of Osteopathic Medicine (now part of Rowan University), where she also completed her internship and residency in the field of family medicine. She has received numerous awards throughout her career, including the Alan A. Gartzman Memorial Award for excellence during her residency, and has served on various committees. In 2015, she was elected to the executive board of the North Carolina Osteopathic Medical Association as their membership chair and was selected to be an official speaking ambassador for the American Osteopathic Association, representing the state of North Carolina in addressing relevant issues in health and wellness.

She is a member of the American Osteopathic Association, North Carolina Osteopathic Medical Association, Obesity Medicine Association, American College of Osteopathic Family Physicians, North Carolina Society for the American College of Osteopathic Family Physicians, National Medical Association, National Osteopathic Medical Association and the Christian Medical and Dental Association.

<u>Personal Reflections</u>

_____

_____

_____

_____

_____

_____

_____

_____

_____

_____

_____

_____

_____

_____

Personal Reflections

_____

_____

_____

_____

_____

_____

_____

_____

_____

_____

_____

_____

_____

_____

_____

<u>Personal Reflections</u>

_____

_____

_____

_____

_____

_____

_____

_____

_____

_____

_____

_____

Dr. Tiffany Lowe-Payne

Made in the USA
Charleston, SC
05 April 2016